Benjamin Jesty

Dorset's Vaccination Pioneer

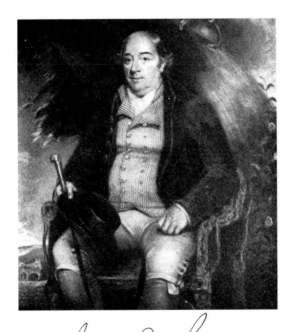

Patrick J Pead

Time*f*ile Books

Time*f*ile Books
a Division of
Patrick J Pead
Chichester
West Sussex

First published in Great Britain
by Time*f*ile Books on 26th October 2009
Commemorating the 30th anniversary
of the global eradication of smallpox

A catalogue record for this book
is available from the British Library

ISBN 978-0-9551561-1-3

Printed and bound in Great Britain by
Selsey Press Ltd
West Sussex
England

Contents

Illustrations

Introduction

During 1985, a chance encounter with an intriguing inscription on a gravestone in the churchyard of St Nicholas of Myra at Worth Matravers near Swanage, led me to research the life of a Dorset farmer named Benjamin Jesty. This resulted in my establishing the location of the world's first authenticated vaccination and discovering Jesty's 'long-lost' portrait. Both findings are significant in the history of medicine. The purpose of this booklet is to provide a brief overview of my investigations. I hope it will introduce the reader to a remarkable gentleman who should inspire us all. He shows that 'ordinary' people are sometimes capable of extra-ordinary achievements. Jesty deserves more recognition than history has so far bestowed.

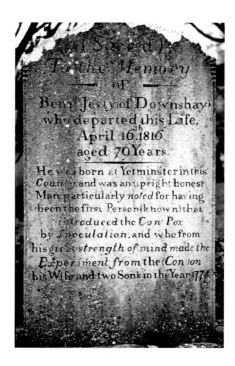

The inscription on the headstone of Benjamin Jesty
as I first saw it in 1985

Smallpox

The origins of vaccination are associated with the disease of smallpox. This dreadful virus infection was a global problem and widespread in Britain in the 18th century when Jesty lived. Epidemics occurred regularly and the young were particularly vulnerable. Estimates suggest that more people died from smallpox than from any other infectious disease in the history of our planet. It was extremely easy to catch the infection through direct contact with a case, or with fomites *i.e.* objects that had been contaminated, or simply by breathing air carrying virus particles. Smallpox is a member of the *Poxviridae*. Measuring some 300 millionths of a millimetre, this microbe is the largest of the viruses that infect humans.

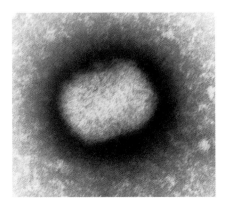

A smallpox virus seen under the electronmicroscope
This particle has been magnified 80,000 times

There were two clinical forms of smallpox. The severe type *Variola major* had a fatality rate of 20 – 50% whereas mild infections with *Variola minor* resulted in death of only 1- 2% of cases. After an incubation period of about 12 days the patient would develop a fever and headache. Two days later a red macular rash appeared on the skin, mostly on the extremities of the body. The areas of rash became raised papules and then developed into blisters of clear fluid which contained virus. The fluid clouded to form pustules that would dry to become crusts.

These dropped off after a while leaving scars on the skin where the lesions had been. People who survived an attack of smallpox often bore these scars for the rest of their lives. Pockmarks on the face were a common sight. Other consequences of infection could include blindness, brain damage, infertility or disfigurement.

Protective measures before vaccination

Until the early 1700s attempts to treat smallpox in Britain were mere quackery. Families were advised to keep patients in a room painted red, or in the dark. They were exposed to extremes of heat and cold. Bleeding was common, as were treatments with vomits and purges. Not surprisingly, none of this had the slightest beneficial effect on the outcome of the disease. However, some countries in the Far East were way ahead of Europe, and had adopted a means of preventing infection centuries earlier.

It must have been noticed in ancient times that people who survived some diseases did not seem to be prone to them later in life. Thucydides noted this in 430 BC when writing about the plague of Athens. Someone in the Orient must have deduced that a similar magical protection might follow if a 'morsel' of the disease was deliberately given to a recipient, because a method came into practise in China, Tibet and India to achieve this. Crusts were collected from the skin of mild cases of smallpox. These were ground into a powder and administered by blowing the material through a tube into the nasal passage of a recipient. This process is termed insufflation.

As the procedure became used more widely it was modified. The Persians preferred to ingest the powder. In Turkey, smallpox material was rubbed into a cut in the skin made by a small needle. This Turkish 'ingrafting' procedure was observed by two doctors, a Greek named Pylarini and an Italian, Timoni. In the early 1700s they both brought the practice to the notice of the Royal Society in England, but their letters were ignored. When Lady Mary Wortley Montagu accompanied her ambassador husband Edward to Constantinople in 1717 she took a great interest in the technique - with good reason. Her brother had died of smallpox and she had survived an attack in England after being close to death. In 1718 she asked the embassy surgeon Charles Maitland to ingraft her young son. When the Montagus returned to London in 1721 Lady Mary found the capital overrun with smallpox, so she persuaded Maitland to repeat the use of the Turkish method to protect her three-year-old daughter. The Montagus were prominent members of the Court of George 1st and soon there was gossip about this extraordinary event. Lady Mary's friend, Caroline of Ansbach (the Princess of Wales) became interested. She asked for an experiment to be performed on six condemned prisoners in Newgate in order to determine the effect and safety of the procedure. After a further experiment on six charity-children she arranged for her own children to be inoculated. Soon the technique became known in Britain as 'the inoculation'. It was popular amongst the gentry and was taken up by many doctors and apothecaries. Unfortunately, they did not use the simple Turkish method, but prescribed a preparation for recipients that included a meagre, low protein diet for several weeks, accompanied by bleeding and purging. There was no control over the type of smallpox inoculum used and inevitably there were fatalities. The other problem was that inoculation spread smallpox into areas where it had previously been absent. Common folk were less keen on the practice and often received money from the local vestry authorities to encourage them to undergo the procedure.

The inoculation was used throughout the 18th and early 19th centuries until 1840 when it was discontinued in favour of vaccination. Certainly many lives were saved at a time when there was no alternative means of protection, but the hazards of infecting with live smallpox could bring problems, both for recipients and their contacts. Despite this, the principle of the procedure did provide the basis for what was to follow, so inoculation was a very important step in the progress towards the methods of inducing immunity that we have today.

The Yetminster farmer

Inoculation was well established by the time that a baby, Benjamin, was born to Robert and Edith Justy at Winterhayes

Farm near Yetminster. The seventh of eight children, he was baptised at St Andrew's Church on the 19th August 1736. His father is listed as a butcher, but Robert Justy also farmed livestock as his own father had done. Benjamin grew up in the village and probably attended Boyle's School, founded in 1697 with a legacy from Robert Boyle to his servant John Warr for that purpose. After leaving school Benjamin followed his father and other members of his family into farming. At some point he changed his surname to Jesty. The reason for this is not known. Possibly he felt it was logical to use the phonetic spelling of his surname because it fitted the 'Jasty' pronunciation in the Dorset dialect. His signature as Jesty is recorded in 1763 when he was a witness to a marriage, on a document in 1769, and at his own wedding in 1770. The majority of the family, both in Dorset and Somerset, adopted this change of name around the same time.

Benjamin married Elizabeth Notley who lived in nearby Longburton. They raised a total of four sons and three daughters, but had three children at the time of Jesty's vaccination 'experiment', Robert aged 3, Benjamin 2, and infant Betty. The family lived at a farmhouse named 'Upbury' in Church Street, Yetminster. There are many houses of historic importance in the village, but Upbury is the oldest, dating back to medieval times. The central village location is not unusual. It was customary for a

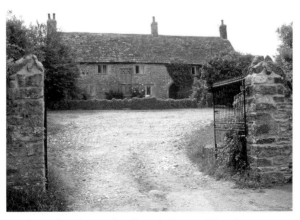

Upbury farmhouse in Church Street, Yetminster
Jesty was living here in 1774

farmhouse to be situated thus, with the associated land scattered around the periphery. Benjamin became a member of the Yetminster Vestry. At this time there were no local authority services as we know them today. Vestries filled this role in rural areas, dealing with every aspect of parish life. Some were functioning from as far back as the 16th century and many detailed records still exist. Most of the duties of the Yetminster Vestry were concerned with provision for the poor – housing, money for clothing, health and burials etc. Jesty was appointed as an Overseer of the Poor and was involved with their health care as part of the Vestry committee. This included making arrangements for inoculations, together with payments to those agreeing to take part. He would have known the local doctors and apothecaries personally and been aware of the hazards of the inoculation procedure.

The cowpox notion

Yetminster lies at the edge of the Blackmore Vale, the place that Thomas Hardy described as 'the vale of the little dairies'. Jesty was a dairy farmer and cattle breeder. He would have been aware of the folklore of cowpox and the notion that it was somehow able to protect people against smallpox. Cowpox is a member of the *Poxvirus* family. It has a structure similar to smallpox and shares some antigenic components with that virus, being capable of stimulating an immune response in humans to both smallpox and cowpox. Country people could easily identify the infection in cows by observing the lesions on the teats of the udders. The disease did not seem to affect the cattle in any other way, but farmers were usually secretive about cowpox, not wishing to lose the sale of their milk and butter products. Those who milked or handled the lesions of cowpox-infected cattle could acquire an infection in the course of their work.

The effect of cowpox on a human was to cause a very mild fever with one or more lesions appearing on the hands where the virus had entered and reproduced in the cells of the outer layers of the skin. All viruses need living cells in order to multiply – their inherent DNA or RNA enters a cell and 'programs' the normal cellular mechanisms to manufacture large numbers of those components which are necessary to form new viruses. When fully mature particles are assembled they emerge from the cell, usually killing it in the process. In humans the cowpox lesion eventually subsides, leaving a scar. During this time the *Poxvirus* antigens have caused the immune system to become activated, and the exposure to cowpox results in a defence against future infection with smallpox.

Dairymaids were noted for their fair complexions. These women usually acquired cowpox in the course of their work and were free of the permanent facial scarring that most smallpox survivors bore as a reminder of the disease.

The first vaccination

Smallpox had returned to Dorset again in the spring of 1774 and Yetminster was threatened with the dread disease. Jesty had acquired cowpox whilst working with cattle in his youth. His notion of cowpox preventing smallpox was strengthened through discussion with two of his dairymaids, Anne Notley and Mary Reade. Both had been infected with cowpox as a result of milking cows. Neither of them had contracted smallpox thereafter, even when nursing relatives with the disease. Jesty was convinced that the folklore was true. Faced with the awful implications of his family suffering the ravages of smallpox, and knowing the hazards of inoculation, he conceived an ingenious idea. Why not use the inoculation procedure but substitute the smallpox material with cowpox? Although this may seem to be an obvious modification to us, in 1774 it represented a quantum leap in thinking.

Confident that he had thought of a safe way to protect his family, Jesty took his wife and two sons to a farm where he knew some cows had the marks of cowpox on their udders. These cattle were owned by a farmer named Elford and were grazing near the neighbouring village of '*Chittenhall*' – the Dorset dialect pronunciation of Chetnole. Jesty had equipped himself with a stocking needle before setting out. This type of needle was widely used for the hand knitting of hose in the area around Sturminster Newton and other parts of Dorset. Here, the local craft remained a thriving cottage industry, in contrast to machine knitting which had been introduced in some Midland counties. Jesty's wife came from nearby Longburton. She would have learnt the traditional skills in her youth and most certainly knitted knee length stockings for her husband with such needles. The slender point would have pierced skin easily.

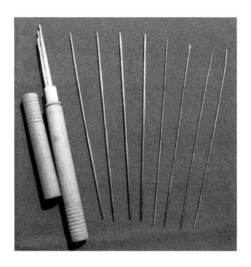

A set of stocking needles
They are six inches in length and pointed at both ends

On reaching the herd, Jesty searched their teats for signs of cowpox. He took material from a lesion onto the tip of a stocking needle and transferred this to his wife's arm, inserting it into her skin immediately below the elbow. He then repeated this for Robert and Benjamin, making punctures just above the elbow in each case. Jesty's venture came to light when a problem arose. Signs of inflammation appeared at the site of Elizabeth's vaccination. Medical assistance was summoned immediately from nearby Cerne – both Mr Henry Meech and Dr Trowbridge are mentioned in the records. Jesty told them about his cowpox experiment. Trowbridge replied, 'You have done a bold thing, but I will get you through if I can', and he treated Elizabeth's condition as a fever. She recovered completely, but knowledge of the vaccinations was no longer confined to the family.

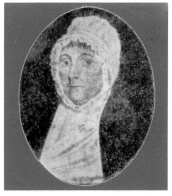
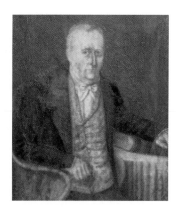

Elizabeth Jesty   Robert Jesty

Word spread throughout the locality and Jesty's deed became well known through gossip in the medical, farming and ecclesiastical fraternities. He became the object of scorn and derision, suffering verbal and physical abuse for some time afterwards when he attended markets. Many regarded him as an inhuman brute. Country people were very suspicious of anything which seemed alien to their traditional beliefs. The last execution for witchcraft had taken place only 62 years before. Jesty steadfastly continued with his parish duties, ignoring the unwelcome attention. The trio of vaccinees remained free of smallpox for the rest of their lives, though often exposed to epidemics of the disease. The two sons were inoculated with smallpox by Dr Trowbridge in 1789. Robert, then aged 18 years, and Benjamin, 17 years, were unaffected, showing that they had developed immunity to the virus.

Keen to establish the exact location of Jesty's historic event, I sought advice from the Hundred of Yetminster Local History Society. Mrs Nina Hayward replied and sent me a list of field names that had been associated with the local Elford family in the eighteenth century. I searched the Yetminster Court records at the Dorset Archives Service and confirmed that four of the listed field names were associated with the farmer, William Elford, at the time of Jesty's vaccinations. The tradition of naming fields goes back at least to medieval times, and names

13

are sometimes derived from Latin or Old English. It was no surprise to find field names linked with the Elfords entered on a Tithe Map of Chetnole drawn seventy years later. I noted that some adjoining fields shown on the map below shared the same names. Most of the field boundaries can still be traced on the current Ordnance Survey Explorer Map of the area. These pastures are in close proximity to a property known as Foys in Chetnole village, which lies 3.7 km (2.3 miles) from the home of Benjamin Jesty. William Elford Snr. lived at 'Napiers' – now 'The Grange' - with his wife, Mary. They had four sons, one being named John Foy Elford. Mary is also mentioned in connection with Foys in the Deeds of the Elford family.

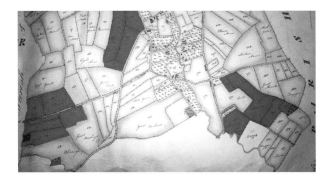

Fields on a Tithe map at the southern extremity of Chetnole
The shaded areas are fields associated with William Elford in 1774
or mentioned in a later sale of his estate

Primed with this information I went to Chetnole to explore the location of the world's first vaccination. Elford's fields are set between the wooded slopes of Melbury Bubb and The Knoll, bisected by the River Wriggle. This landscape has changed little since Jesty's day; the Yeovil/Dorchester railway track being the obvious exception. Whilst taking time to absorb the scenery I realised I could barely see the tower of St Andrew's Church in distant Yetminster away to the north. The material reality of the map measurement brought a new perspective to the situation. The distance from Upbury to Elford's fields bears witness to the extent of Jesty's foresight and planning. What happened here was no fleeting daydream of some country bumpkin; it required inspiration and a firm resolve.

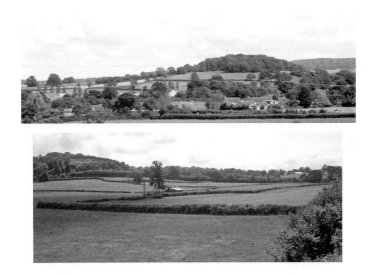

Views of fields in the area of Chetnole shown on the Tithe Map
Benjamin Jesty came here with his wife and two sons in 1774
to vaccinate them with cowpox taken on a stocking needle
from the teats of infected cows owned by William Elford

The outcome of Jesty's *'bold thing'* was that he became reviled by the local population. Learning that of one of their number had introduced matter from a beast of the field into the body of a human being would have evoked strong moral and religious taboos (Exodus 22, 19 '..man shall not… contaminate the form of the Creator with the brute'). The prejudice against Jesty was carried to such a height that a surgeon (possibly Trowbridge) 'almost lost his practice' from following up the results of the experiment. Jesty paid a high price for his ingenuity. Undaunted, he valiantly continued his farming business and attended to his parish duties in the face of a constant atmosphere of abhorrence and suspicion. He did nothing to publicise the merits of his experiment and refrained from conducting further vaccinations whilst living in Yetminster.

Dr Edward Jenner

At this point it is necessary to digress from the story of Jesty in order to place Dr Edward Jenner in context. Jenner is generally regarded as the 'discoverer' of vaccination. He was born on the 17th May 1749 to Stephen Jenner, vicar of Berkeley in Gloucestershire, and his wife Sarah. Both parents died when Edward was aged five so he lived with his eldest sister Mary until she married. At this time he began his schooling at Clissold's boarding school in Wotton-under-Edge. Whilst he was there he suffered the rigours of inoculation performed by Holbrow - a local apothecary who subjected him to the English procedure described previously. Forcibly restrained in the school's inoculation stables, the trauma of this event affected him for years afterwards. The young boy's health deteriorated and he was grossly unhappy, so after only one year at Clissold's he was sent to study as a private student with Dr John Washbourne at Cirencester. Edward was fascinated by natural history but was not considered sufficiently academically equipped for university. In 1763 he was apprenticed to the apothecary Daniel Ludlow in the village of Chipping Sodbury for seven years. During this time he learnt of the cowpox notion from a dairymaid.

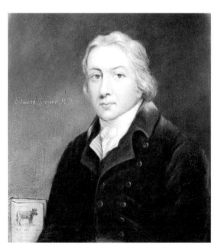

Dr Edward Jenner

After completing his apprenticeship, he paid to study medicine under the great surgeon John Hunter in London and they became good friends. Hunter invited him to stay on as a partner, but in 1773 Jenner decided to follow the career of a country doctor and returned to establish a practice in Berkeley. He did not leave London with a medical degree; this was purchased for him from the University of St. Andrews by some friends much later in 1792.

At the age of forty Edward married Catherine Kingscote who was a niece of the Countess of Suffolk. Her father was rich and connected to the nobility. They moved into The Chantry in Berkeley, which is now the home of The Jenner Museum.

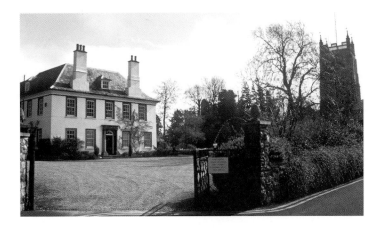

The Chantry in Berkeley
The tower of St Mary the Virgin Church is to the right

Part of Jenner's services as rural general practioner was to provide inoculation. Jenner used a method developed by Daniel Sutton which involved the application of a small inoculum of smallpox material without the trauma of the weakening diet and the bleeding *etc*. Jenner's interest in the cowpox notion was rekindled through his inoculation of people in the local farming community who failed to react, and who told him that they had previously acquired cowpox in the course of their work. He made notes about this and also a condition of horses known as 'grease'. Jenner proposed that cowpox was

17

derived from grease by transmission from horse to cattle by farm hands. He persisted with this idea even when publishing his vaccination findings. The concept was flawed and brought him much criticism later.

Jenner discussed his interest in the protective nature of cowpox many times with his medical friends - so much so that they tired of it. However, his neighbour Fewster had read a paper to the London Medical Society in 1765 on 'Cowpox and its ability to Prevent Smallpox' and this must have strengthened his belief. Fewster did not carry out any experiments because he felt that inoculation was so well understood that he saw no need for a substitute. Jenner had maintained his friendship with Hunter who was always encouraging him to experiment, but he did nothing. This is understandable – he had a lot to lose - his reputation as a doctor was well established by now, and he had been made a Fellow of The Royal Society in 1789 for his research on the natural history of the cuckoo. The idea of actually transferring material from a cow into a human must have raised the same taboos that surfaced in Jesty's time, and it was a risk that he clearly would not undertake lightly.

In the early autumn of 1794 Jenner became very ill. Typhus is mentioned in contemporary accounts but it is now thought that some other infection, possibly typhoid fever, caused his health to suffer. He remained weak into the spring of the following year when his medical advisors suggested a period of recuperation in Cheltenham. Catherine, Edward and their two infants arrived in this fashionable spa town where social amenities abounded in the wake of royal patronage. After he regained his health, the family's stay in Cheltenham was to bring Jenner into contact with those in the higher echelons of society. These included intellectuals and influential members of the professions from far and wide. He enjoyed conversation, making many friends and useful contacts during his time there.

The family returned to Berkeley in the autumn of 1795. Something must have given Jenner a new-found confidence to proceed further with his interest in protection against smallpox, for he performed his first vaccination experiment on the 14th May 1796. Using a lancet he took cowpox material from a lesion on the hand of a dairymaid, Sarah Nelmes, and transferred it by skin incision to the arm of an eight-year-old boy named James Phipps - a person to person vaccination. Jenner then inoculated Phipps with smallpox on the 1st July and found that he was unaffected. The following year he wrote an account of the experiment and showed it to Sir Joseph Banks and Everard Home of The Royal Society. He was advised that it would be rejected for publication because it contained too little evidence to support his claims. Jenner carried out a further series of experiments in 1798. This time he began by taking cowpox from the udder of a cow, as Jesty had done 24 years before, and transferred it to the arm of a boy named William Summers. He then waited until a lesion appeared on Summers's skin before he took material from this lesion and vaccinated another boy, William Pead. He followed this by a sequence of at least six further human to human transfers in children before inoculating two of them with smallpox to show that they were protected.

Now Jenner decided to publish without risking the possibility of refusal. He paid for the paper to be printed by Sampson Low at Berwick Street in London. Its title was '*An Inquiry into The Causes and Effects of the Variolae Vaccinae, a disease discovered in some of the Western Counties of England particularly Gloucestershire and known by the name of The Cowpox*'. Within the text he actually uses the word 'virus', though his meaning in ignorance of microbes was 'a poison'. His derivation of *Variolae Vaccinae* was from the Latin for 'smallpox of the cow'.

This was the pivotal event in Jenner's professional life. After an initial lack of interest, evidence began to appear in support of his claims. Progress was entirely due to Jenner's persistence and the support he solicited from notable men of the day. The protective effect of natural cowpox infection in humans was confirmed by other doctors. Vaccinations by Drs Woodville and Pearson took place in London when a fresh supply of cowpox lymph became available in 1799. Inoculation with smallpox was still in common use, so there was ample opportunity to use this to challenge the cowpox-vaccinated subjects for evidence of protection. Vaccine lymph was soon distributed throughout England and was sent to interested practitioners in some other European countries. Jenner's published work was confirmed in writing by others over the next few decades. He generated a group of enthusiastic supporters, though he also faced opposition from some of his contemporaries who were in receipt of remuneration for their inoculation services. Within three years the *Inquiry* had been translated into French, German, Italian, Dutch, Spanish and Latin. Arm-to-arm transfer of vaccine was maintained in Britain until 1898.

Had Jenner kept his vaccination method secret it is very likely that he would have amassed a personal fortune. Instead, he chose to make his knowledge freely available, and worked hard to encourage others to adopt the technique. He was awarded two substantial sums of money from the Government in recognition of this - £10,000 in 1802 and a further £20,000 in 1807. He was not rewarded for being the first to use the procedure. If his petition had rested solely on having been the first to vaccinate with cowpox it could not have been upheld. Jenner received honours from many countries of the world and became the most decorated man of his generation. He was introduced to those in the highest strata of society including some of the crowned heads of Europe, but he was never given a knighthood. His wife's long battle with illness eventually took its toll. Catherine Jenner died in September 1815. Her husband was to survive her for another eight years. He died on 26th January 1823 after being copiously bled following 'a fit of apoplexy' (a stroke). James Phipps was among the mourners at his funeral on the 3rd February. Jenner lies next to Catherine, beside the altar in The Minster Church of St Mary the Virgin in Berkeley,

Inoculation and Vaccination

There is a considerable volume of literature on the origins of vaccination and it is easy to become confused over the terminology. Some clarification is needed.

Inoculation - the deliberate infection of a person with live smallpox virus collected from the skin lesions of a patient suffering from the mild form of the disease. Infection was achieved by seeding superficial incisions made in the recipient's skin with a lancet. Either fresh smallpox lymph or powder prepared from dried scabs was used. It was banned in 1840.

Vaccination – the deliberate transfer of cowpox virus to a human, by insertion into the skin using one of a number of types of needle or a lancet. The virus was contained in lymph collected from a lesion on the udder or teat of a cow that displayed typical signs of cowpox. Vaccination is sometimes referred to as 'inoculation for (*i.e. with*) the cowpox' in old books and documents.

The word 'vaccination' was coined in 1803 by one of Jenner's friends, Richard Dunning, a naval surgeon living in Plymouth. Its derivation is from the latin word *vacca* – the cow, so the literal interpretation of vaccination is 'from the cow'.

The British Government introduced compulsory vaccination for infants in 1853. This led to a voluble and well-organised anti-vaccinationist movement led by John Gibbs. Its ranks included eminent doctors, clergymen and Members of Parliament. Many were prepared to go to prison in defence of their beliefs. Compulsion was ended by the 1898 Act, which provided a 'conscience clause' and this Act was strengthened by another in 1907. This is how the term 'conscientious objector' entered the English language. By the end of the 19th century Louis Pasteur had developed his 'germ theory' and produced immunising preparations for anthrax and rabies. He suggested they be called vaccines in honour of Jenner.

Jesty's move to Purbeck

We can now return to the story of Benjamin Jesty. The Rev Morgan Jones, the rector of Ryme Intrinseca near Yetminster, also had a living at Worth Matravers in Purbeck. He told Jesty of a vacant tenancy of a farm near Harmans Cross, not far from Swanage. This tenancy was at Downshay Manor; the farm was larger and the accommodation more spacious than Upbury. Jesty moved there with his family during March 1796, just before Jenner carried out his first vaccination in the same year. Benjamin and Elizabeth now had a total of seven children and they must have considered that Downshay was more suitable for the larger family.

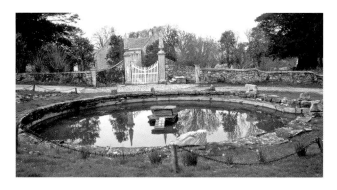

Downshay Manor – previously Dunshay – near Harman's Cross

The house is hidden away in a small valley where time seems to have stood still. The driveway descends through trees and banks of wild flowers to widen out into a cobbled courtyard with a central pond. The house is roughly square on plan but has been subject to alteration over the centuries. Two gables flank a central porch on the east front. The north wing was in ruins in Jesty's time but was rebuilt in 1906. Having settled the family into their new home, Jesty resumed his farming activities.

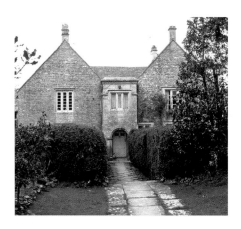

Downshay - the north wing (right) has been rebuilt

There is evidence that a Benjamin Jesty performed more vaccinations after moving to Purbeck. A man named Bykur wrote to the *Southern Times* in 1902 about a conversation he had with 'an aged villager, who unquestionably was vaccinated, with others, by Jesty personally when at Downshay farm'. In the church at nearby Worth Matravers there is a memorial to a Mary Brown, whose daughter Abigail 'was personally inoculated for the cow pox by Benjamin Jesty of Downshay'. Whether the practitioner was Benjamin senior or junior is not known.

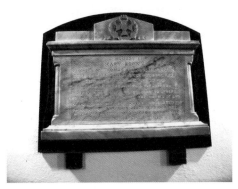

Memorial to May Brown in the church at Worth Matravers mentioning Jesty's vaccination of her daughter Abigail

In the spring of 1803 Jesty met the Rev Andrew Bell. Dr Bell was a celebrated man of letters who had distinguished himself in India, where he set up a self-help scheme of primary education for orphan children. On his return to England in 1801 he was appointed to the livings of Swanage and Worth Matravers where he hoped to enjoy some years of restful vocation. It was now twenty-nine years since Jesty had vaccinated his family. By this time, Dr Edward Jenner had published his vaccination experiments in his *'Inquiry'*. Dr Bell had become an enthusiastic vaccinator and was dismayed to find that the efficacy of vaccination was still doubted by many living in the Isle of Purbeck. He brought some vaccine material from Edinburgh and started a campaign to popularise it immediately.

The clergyman's account of his meeting with Jesty is set down in great detail by the author Robert Southey in his biography *The Life of the Rev Andrew Bell* and is the closest we are able to get to the first vaccinator's own version of events. Bell felt that the extraordinary deeds of 1774 'may be thought not unworthy of a place in the history of the cow-pox. If it should have any influence with those parents who decline the offer made to them of having their children vaccinated, my object is attained; and let Mr Jesty have that share of credit'. Unaware of Pearson's petition for Jesty during the 1802 debate at the Commons Committee, Bell wrote letters to him in 1803 and 1804. The rector was so impressed with the farmer and the story of his enterprise that, on Sunday the 15th July 1806, he preached the same sermon twice in honour of the man 'whose discovery of the efficacy of the cowpock against smallpox is so often forgotten by those who have heard of Dr Jenner'.

The invitation to London

Soon after Bell's intercession, Benjamin Jesty received a letter dated 25th July 1805. It was an invitation to visit London. This came from the secretary of the Original Vaccine Pock Institution, Will Sancho. The Vaccine Pock Institution had been founded on the 2nd December 1799 at Warwick Street, near Charing Cross. The organisation moved to 'a more commodious house' at 5 Golden Square in April 1801, then finally on to Broad Street at its junction with Poland Street.

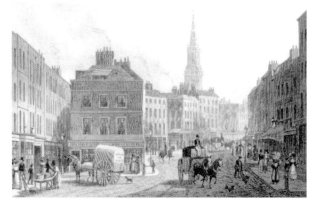

Engraving showing Broad Street in Georgian London
(the Vaccine Pock Institution was the tall building at extreme right)

Jesty accepted the invitation and called upon his neighbour, the father of the Rev J.M.Colson, to borrow some saddle-bags for the transport of clean shirts. He was promptly advised that saddlebags would be considered '*extinctum genus*' in the City. Colson senior supplied him with a portmanteau as a more suitable and convenient vehicle. Benjamin's family tried to persuade him that he should attire himself more fashionably but to no avail. He exclaimed that 'he did not see why he should dress better in London than in the country' and accordingly wore his usual clothing, which was rather old-fashioned. Jesty mounted his horse and was accompanied on this three day journey by his eldest son, Robert , then 28 years old.

The two Dorset men met with much attention from the members of the society, who were greatly amused by Benjamin's manners and appearance. Jesty was not enthusiastic about the metropolis, but admitted the one great comfort was that he could be shaved every day instead of wearing a beard from Saturday to Saturday. Normally he would only shave before attending the weekly market in Wareham. The physicians, surgeons and apothecaries of the Institution questioned Jesty about his vaccination 'experiment', listened to his reasoning, and received permission for Robert to be publicly inoculated with live smallpox in order to prove he was still protected against the disease. Jesty had developed a plausible hypothesis for vaccination with cowpox out of his conversations with the milkmaids at Upbury – an idea deduced from his own observations and the application of rural logic. This is made clear in the answers he gave when examined by the officials of the Institute in August 1805. Twelve of the Institute's examining officers were signatories to a statement commemorating the 'antivariolus efficacy' of Jesty's cowpox vaccinations. This was issued from their establishment at No. 44 Broad Street in London on the 6th September 1805 and published in the *Edinburgh Medical and Surgical Journal* soon after. Their statement is reproduced here as a direct transcription from the original publication, with the exception of the letter 's', which appears as 'f' in the document.

'Mr Benjamin Jesty, farmer of Downshay, in the Isle of Purbeck, having (agreeably to an invitation from the Medical Establishment of the Original Vaccine Pock Institution, Broad Street, Golden Square) visited London in August 1805 to communicate certain facts relating to the Cow Pock Institution, we think it a matter of justice to himself, and beneficial to the public, to attest that, among other facts, he has afforded decisive evidence of his having vaccinated his wife and two sons, Robert and Benjamin, in the year 1774; who were thereby rendered unsusceptible of the small-pox, as appears from the exposure of all the three parties to that disorder frequently during the course of 31 years, and from the inoculation of the two sons for the small-pox fifteen years ago. That he was led to undertake this novel practice in 1774, to counteract the small-pox, at that time prevalent at Yetminster, where he then resided, from knowing the common opinion of the country, ever since he was a boy (now 60 years ago), that persons who had gone through the cow-pock naturally, *i.e.* by taking it from cows, were unsusceptible of the small-pox; by himself being incapable of taking the small-pox, having gone through the cow-pock many years before; from having personally known many individuals, who, after the cow-pock, could not have the small-pox excited; from believing that the cow-pock was an affection free from danger; and from his opinion that, by the cow-pock inoculation, he should avoid ingrafting various diseases of the human constitution, such as "the Evil, madnes, lues, and many bad humours," as he called them.

The remarkable vigorous health of Mr. Jesty, his wife and two sons, now 31 years subsequent to the cow-pock, and his own healthy appearance, at this time 70 years of age, afford a singularly strong proof of the harmlessness of that affection; but the public must, with particular interest, hear that, during the late visit to town, Mr Robert Jesty very willingly submitted publicly to inoculation for the small-pox in the most rigorous manner; and that Mr. Jesty also was subjected to the trial of inoculation for the cow-pock after the most efficacious mode, without either of them being infected. The circumstances on which Mr. Jesty purposely instituted the vaccine-pock inoculation in his own family, – viz. *without any precedent,* but merely from reasoning upon the

26

nature of the affection among cows, and from knowing its effects in the casual way among men, his exemption from the prevailing popular prejudices, and his disregard of the clamorous reproaches of his neighbours, in our opinion, will entitle him to the respect of the public for his superior strength of mind. But, further, his conduct in again furnishing such decisive proofs of the permanent anti-variolous efficacy of the cow-pock, on the present discontented state of mind in many families, by submitting to inoculation, justly claims at least the gratitude of the country. As a testimony of our personal regard, and to commemorate so extraordinary a fact, as that of preventing the small-pox by inoculating for the cow-pock 31 years ago, at our request, a three quarter length picture of Mr Jesty is painted by that excellent artist Mr Sharp, to be preserved at the Original Vaccine Pock Institution'.

It is understandable that Jesty, a dairy farmer, preferred to take cowpox directly from the cow. His simple explanation is convincing:

'There is little risk in introducing into the human constitution matter from the cow as we already without danger eat the flesh and blood, drink the milk and cover ourselves with the skin of this innocuous animal'

The most likely hazard arising from transferring cowpox lymph directly from a cow's udder to human skin by incision (at a time when there was no concept of microbes or hygienic practice) would have been from contaminating bacteria that might predispose to sepsis spreading from the site of vaccination. This was the most likely cause of Elizabeth's fever.

The portrait of Benjamin Jesty

The Officers of the Vaccine Pock Institution considered the ingenious farmer worthy of recognition. They presented Jesty with a pair of gold mounted lancets, a testimonial scroll, the sum of fifteen guineas for his expenses and most significantly, commissioned his portrait to be painted in oils. The chosen artist was Michael W Sharp, who was patronised by the family of King George IIIrd and whose sitters had included the first Duke of Wellington. His studio at that time was in Great Marlborough

Street, a short distance from the Institute offices in Broad Street. The painting was completed quite quickly whilst Jesty was in London. The farmer proved an impatient sitter and would only sit still when Sharp's wife played to him upon the pianoforte.

Sharp's finished canvas was exhibited at Somerset House before being hung at the Vaccine Pock Institution. When this closed in 1807 the portrait was acquired by the Director, Dr Pearson, and when he died it was given to Robert Jesty. When Robert Jesty died in 1839 the portrait could not be bequeathed to the other recipient of Jesty's vaccination, his second son Benjamin, because he had died the year before. Edith (Robert's widow) gave it to her daughter, Edith, who had been married to Francis Pope for five years. Ownership of the portrait passed out of the Jesty family at this stage. After Edith's death it was inherited by her eldest son Frank Ezekiel Pope. The picture was recorded as hanging at Frank Ezekiel's home, Chilfrome Farm in Dorset, when Dr Edgar Crookshank visited him in 1888. All records of the portrait ceased after this time. A few years ago I decided to investigate whether this portrait still existed, and if so, where it might lie hidden. Research into the genealogies of the Jesty and Pope families yielded a preliminary, but incomplete, provenance. One contact, the late Christopher Pope of the Eldridge-Pope Brewery, told me that he thought he had seen the painting during a visit to relatives in South Africa. Sadly, he became very ill and died before he could help further.

The project was given a boost when I was able to resource some people living in South Africa, who were associated with the Pope family business. Contact was eventually made with the owner of the portrait through an extremely tenuous chain of circumstances; his name was Charles Pope and he was living in the Eastern Cape of South Africa. He knew the story of Jesty and said that the near life-sized portrait was hanging at his family home on a vast farm near Molteno about 180 miles from the coast. Notice of my find was published in 2005. The recovery of this definitive image from the past is a cause for celebration because the picture was thought to be lost and its very existence doubted.

Charles Pope helped me to complete the provenance. Two of Frank Ezekiel's brothers had emigrated to Cape Colony in South Africa in 1858. The sons of one of these brothers served with the South African Heavy Artillery in France during the First World War. One of the soldiers, Francis William Pope, came over to visit his uncle in Dorset during leave from the Front. Frank Ezekiel had no direct heirs, and was so pleased to see his nephew that he left his entire estate to him in his will, including the portrait. Francis returned to Dorset in 1934 to collect the family silver and other valuables from Chilfrome Farm. He found the portrait in a barn. It was damaged and he arranged for it to be repaired in London before taking it back to South Africa. The painting then hung in the Pope family home at Molteno. It was inherited by Francis's son Francis Stanley Pope, and in due course his grandson Charles Pope, whom I contacted in 2004 in a memorable telephone call.

Charles made it clear that he was interested in selling the portrait and placed the sale with an agent in the UK. It was acquired by The Wellcome Trust for the Wellcome Library's collection. Wellcome told me that my publications about Jesty had directly influenced their purchase. Immediately the portrait was returned to England in June 2006 I was invited to London to see it. A programme of restoration began and the canvas was completed in 2007 with a celebratory reception at Wellcome's Gibbs Building in Euston Road in December of that year. The frame restoration was completed in 2008; canvas and frame were then reunited.

The Dorset County Museum accepted a proposal to apply for loan of the painting during 2009 to mark its rediscovery and repatriation. Those involved felt that an exhibition would be a unique historic event for Dorset, being the first public display of the painting since 1805 and a providing a prime opportunity to view the restored picture. The 26th October was chosen as the launch date, coinciding with the 30th anniversary of the initial announcement by the World Health Organisation of the global eradication of smallpox (see below). The painting had returned to Dorset since leaving the county in 1934 having survived a journey halfway round the world. It was immensely rewarding for me to see it in Dorchester. My considerable thanks are owed to the museum authorities, to Wellcome, and to all those who helped to make the exhibition possible. The portrait remains in the ownership of the Wellcome Library and I hope it will be exhibited at other venues in the years to come.

Jesty and Jenner

It is interesting to compare these two men, a humble farmer largely forgotten by history until recent times, and the world famous doctor. Edward Jenner was a controversial figure, being portrayed by his supporters as a saintly genius or described by his detractors as a social climber who sought fame and status. There were immense differences in their social standing, associated with the advantages and disadvantages of their professions; yet their individual approaches to making vaccination a practical measure show some similarity.

Both knew about the horrors of smallpox and were motivated to do something about it. Both were given the cowpox notion by dairymaids and saw the potential of using cowpox as a safer alternative to smallpox for inoculation. Both were prepared to put their ideas into practice and were exposed to ridicule for their actions.

Their places in history have been determined by the ability to bring the new development to the attention of others by publication, and to follow this with further evidence in order to convince them of its benefits. Jesty was clearly not able to present an account of his experiment in writing and would have been ignored by the medical profession if he had. The local doctors who knew what he had done were aware of the abhorrence expressed by people around them and distanced themselves until later, when several wrote letters confirming the Chetnole event. Jenner was able to discuss his theories with colleagues and carry out further experiments to prove them. Despite the rejection of his initial report, Jenner's situation enabled him to publish his findings and persuade the world that he had found something which would greatly benefit mankind. Faced with the same ignorance and derision that Jesty had experienced a quarter of a century earlier, Jenner realised that he had to use his influential medical and social contacts to overcome disbelief and sometimes outright opposition. Jesty had no-one to assist him and must have felt that it was unwise and pointless to try to convince others.

Whether Jenner knew of Jesty's experiment, or those performed by others who used cowpox before 1796, is unknown. Certainly there is no written record that he was inspired, or given confidence to act after such a long period of reluctance by another user of vaccination proper. However there are two pertinent factors. Much of Jenner's correspondence did not survive after his death, and unlike other famous names in science and medicine Jenner never gave credit to others in his writing. However, he did have several good medical contacts in Dorset and I am still researching this interesting question at the time of writing.

Was Jesty the first vaccinator in 1774?

Fewster drew attention to the protective effects of cowpox in 1765, as did a German bailiff Jobst Bose in 1769, but neither vaccinated. Pulteney received a letter during 1798 from a Bridport surgeon named Downe claiming 'a history of intentional *(cowpox)* inoculation' in 1771. Downe's communication referred to an event involving his father and grandfather. However, this remained unconfirmed by contemporaries, and Crookshank considered the account as not sufficiently reliable to be regarded as authentic. It was not printed in the report of evidence considered by the Commons Committee that debated Edward Jenner's petition. A Dorset doctor, Nash, wrote notes in 1781 recommending cowpox as a superior method of inoculation, but encouraged others to make the experiment. A surgeon named Nicholas Bragge of Axminster, Devon alleged in 1802 that 'It is now more than thirty years ago that I first made experiments, and proved that the vaccine disease was a preservative against the smallpox' but the date is in doubt. Others writing about Bragge estimated time intervals when he 'proved the efficacy' as 1782, and mentioned a failed experiment in 1788. Bragge also implied that a farmer's wife, Mrs Rendall, living near Lyme Regis in Dorset, vaccinated herself and three or four children around 1780. Cowpox *was* used for vaccination in 1791 by Plett and Jensen who lived in Holstein, Bavaria. Jenner began in 1796.

Given the vagaries of the historical record, it seems reasonable to recognise Benjamin Jesty as the first authentic vaccinator. He was validated by independent contemporary sources.

Jesty's gravestone

Benjamin Jesty died on the 16th April 1816, seven years before Jenner. He lies next to his wife in the churchyard of St Nicholas of Myra in Worth Matravers, not far from Swanage in East Dorset. Their graves are to be found at the rear of the church.

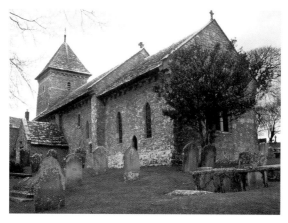

St Nicholas of Myra Church, Worth Matravers

The inscription on his tombstone provides a posthumous publication of his vaccinations and reads:

'(Sacred) To the Memory of Benj.m Jesty, (of Downshay) who departed this Life, April 16th 1816 aged 79 years. He was born at Yetminster in this County, and was an upright honest Man: particularly noted for having been the first Person (known) that introduced the Cowpox by Inoculation, and who from his great strength of mind made the Experiment from the (Cow) on his Wife and two Sons in the Year 1774'

Many people have read this inscription over the past 193 years including several eminent members of the medical profession. When Sir William Osler visited he was accompanied by Professor W R Bett who wrote in 1929 'this epitaph has kept Benjamin Jesty afloat on the stream of time'. Over the years, the condition of the inscription deteriorated to the extent that in 2007 it was hardly readable, and an explanatory notice had been set up at the foot of the grave. During the early part of 2008 the headstones of both Jesty and his wife were cleaned and the lettering was re-cut where necessary, then repainted. This was funded by the Worth Matravers Parochial Church Council, members of the Jesty family and myself. The work was undertaken by two young craftsmen, Mark Haysom and Wayne Monks of Lander's Quarries. A service of rededication of the two memorials was conducted by the Rev Judith Malins on the 16th April 2008, the 192nd anniversary of Jesty's death. We hope that those visiting the peaceful country churchyard in future years by accident or design will read this famous inscription and find a moment to ponder over the implications.

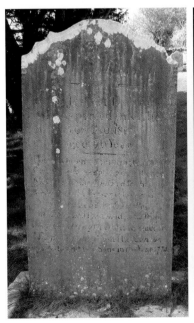 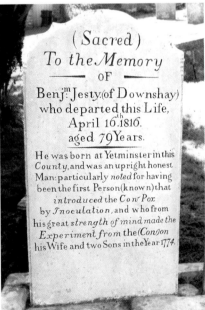

2007   2008
Jesty's headstone before and after restoration

The eradication of smallpox

The World Health Assembly agreed in 1966 to start an eradication programme to free the world from smallpox, and this was launched the following year. At this time, the disease existed in 46 countries with an estimated 10-15 million infections per year, of which 2 million were fatal. The campaign relied upon a principle which became known as 'surveillance-containment' *i.e.* a combination of identification of cases, isolation of patients and mass vaccination. Modern smallpox vaccine contains *vaccinia* virus, not the cowpox virus used by Benjamin Jesty and Edward Jenner. The introduction of the Wyeth 'bifurcated needle' during the campaign simplified the vaccination procedure and its effectiveness improved when centrally produced vaccine was adopted.

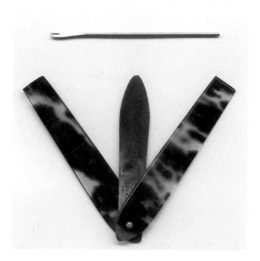

A Wyeth needle (top) as used in the WHO smallpox eradication campaign seen in comparison with a lancet (bottom) similar to those used by doctors and apothecaries for inoculation and early vaccinations

The Wyeth needle measures 5 cms in length – the tines of the bifurcation hold exactly the correct volume when dipped into the vaccine fluid. The vaccine was then applied by a series

Erratum:
Page 35 line 19 '2008' should read '1979'

of rapid insertions into the epidermis of the skin, making the procedure quick and easy for staff with relatively little training. It was ideal for use in areas where more sophisticated facilities did not exist.

The World Health Organisation teams overcame huge difficulties in pursuit of their goal, coping with political problems, wars, floods and famines, a funding crisis, reaching nomadic peoples and those in remote areas with barely sufficient staff. Gradually country after country was freed from the disease until the final *naturally occurring* case was detected in Somalia on the 26th October 1977 – a man named Ali Maow Maalin. He was a hospital cook living in Merca some fifty miles from Mogadishu.

There was no announcement from the WHO of their achievement at that time, which later proved to be fortuitous. Unfortunately the virus was to claim one more victim and contribute to the death of two other people. Janet Parker, a photographer working in the medical school at Birmingham, England, contracted *Variola major* in 2008. She worked on the floor above the microbiology department where smallpox virus was being handled. Her infection was thought to be caused by the inhalation of virus in air from a ventilation duct connecting the floors. Mrs Parker died on the 11th September. Her mother survived an episode of smallpox but her father, who did not have the disease, died of a heart attack. Safety precautions in the microbiology laboratory had been criticised previously, and the head of the department, Professor Henry Bedson, took his own life.

Every country remained free from naturally occurring smallpox after Ali Maalin was diagnosed. After a two year interval came an announcement on the 26th October 1979 by Dr Halfdan Mahler (Director of the WHO) that the disease had been eradicated. The global commission issued a parchment document on the 9th December proclaiming the eradication in six languages signed by those responsible for the magnificent achievement. This was ratified by the World Health Assembly on the 8th May 1980. Thus the 'Speckled Monster', smallpox, which had killed more people than any other infectious disease in history, was defeated over a period of 12 years, 9 months and 26 days.

Bibliography

Baron, J. *The Life of Edward Jenner MD...with Illustrations from His Doctrines, and selections from His Correspondence.* London: H Colburn, 1827.

Baxby, D. *Jenner's Smallpox Vaccine: The Riddle of Vaccinia Virus and its Origin.* London: Heinemann Educational, 1981.

Baxby, D. *Vaccination – Jenner's Legacy.* Berkeley: The Jenner Educational Trust, 1994.

Baxby, D. *Smallpox Vaccine, Ahead of its Time.* Berkeley: The Jenner Museum, 2001.

Bazin H. *The Eradication of Smallpox.* San Diego; London: Academic Press, 2000.

Crookshank, E M. *History and Pathology of Vaccination.* London: H K Lewis, 1889.

Fenner, F, Henderson, D A, Arita, I, Jezak Z, and Ladnyi, I D. *Smallpox and its eradication.* Geneva: World Health Organization, 1988

Fisher, R B. *Edward Jenner 1749-1823.* London: André Deutsch Ltd, 1991.

Fisk, D. *Dr Jenner of Berkeley.* London, William Heinemann, 1959.

Glynn, I and Glynn J. *The Life and Death of Smallpox.* London: Profile Books, 2004.

Gould, G M. 'Medical discoveries by the non-medical' in *JAMA,* Vol 40 (1903), p 1477.

Hammarsten J F, Tattersall W, and Hammarsten J E. 'Who discovered smallpox vaccination? Edward Jenner or Benjamin Jesty?' in *Trans Am Clin Climatol Assoc*, Vol 90 (1979), pp 44 – 55.

Hart, F D. 'Benjamin Jesty, farmer vaccinator'
in *Br J Clin Pract*, Vol 42 (1988), pp 33 – 34.

Haviland, A. 'The proto-martyr to vaccination'
in *Lancet*, Vol 2 (1862), p 291.

Hopkins, D R. *Princes and Peasants: Smallpox in History.*
Chicago and London: University of Chicago, 1983.

Horton, G C. 'Jabs'
in *London Rev Books*, Vol 14 (1992), pp 22 – 23.

Horton, G C. 'Myths in medicine'
in *British Medical Journal*, Vol. 310 (1995), p 62.

Jenner E. *An Inquiry into the Causes and Effects of the Variolae Vaccinae, a Disease.....and known by the name of the Cow Pox.*
London: Sampson Low, 1798.

Jenner, G C. *The evidence at large, as laid before the committee of the House of Commons, respecting Dr Jenner's discovery of vaccine inoculation, together with the debate: and some observations on the contravening evidence.* London: J Murray, 1805.

Katscher, F. 'Pioneers of vaccination'
in *Nature*, Vol 381 (1996), pp 468 – 469.

Kilpatrick, D C. 'Farmer Jesty and the discovery of vaccination'
in *J Clin Pathol*, Vol 46 (1993) p 287.

Machin, R. *The Houses of Yetminster.*
Bristol: University of Bristol, 1978.

McCrae, T. 'Benjamin Jesty: a pre-Jennerian vaccinator'
in *Johns Hopkins Hosp Bull*, Vol 11 (1900), pp 42 – 44.

O'M, J (no surname) 'The Original Vaccine Inoculator'
in *A Medical Bulletin*, Vol II (1954), pp 129 – 139.
Published by May & Baker Ltd

Pead, P J. 'Benjamin Jesty: new light in the dawn of vaccination'
in *Lancet*, Vol 362 (2003), pp 2104 – 2109.

Pead, P J. 'The first vaccinators 'lost' portrait is found'
in *Wellcome History*, Issue 30 (2006), p 7.

Pead, P J. *Vaccination Rediscovered*
Chichester, Sussex, Timefile Books, 2006.   (*now out of print*)

Pearson, G. *An Inquiry concerning the history of the cowpox,
principally with a view to supersede and extinguish the smallpox.*
London: J. Johnson, 1798.

Pearson G *et al.* 'Report of The Original Vaccine Pock Institution'
in *Edin Med Surg J*, Vol 1, No. 4 (1805), pp 513 – 514.

Plett, P C. 'Peter Plett und die ubrigen Entdecker der
Kuhpockenimpfung vor Edward Jenner'
in *Sudhoffs Archiv*, Vol 90 - 2 (2006), pp 219 – 232.

Razzell, P. *The Conquest of Smallpox.*
Firle, Sussex: Caliban Books, 1977.

Saunders, P. *Edward Jenner, The Cheltenham Years.*
Hanover and London: University Press of New England, 1982.

Southey, C C. *The Life of the Rev Andrew Bell.*
London: John Murray, 1844.

The History of Inoculation and Vaccination.
Lecture Memoranda XVIIth International Congress of Medicine
Burroughs Wellcome & Co, 1913.

Wallace, M. *The First Vaccinator.*
Wareham and Swanage: Anglebury-Bartlett, 1981.

Note: there is much more bibliography on this topic. The references quoted here are only those used for this booklet.